Qooba (Dermatophytosis)

Dr.Adnan Mastan

BUMS, MD (Medicine),

FIII, DHI, DHM

Dedicated to

Prof. Rais-ur-Rahman

for his constant encouragement and support

CONTENTS

QOOBA/DERMATOPHYTOSIS

SYNONYMS:

Persian: Paryun

Hindi: Daad

English: Ringworm, Dermatophytosis, Superficial Dermatomycosis, Jungle Rot, Tineasis.

DEFINITION

Qooba (Dermatophytosis) is a roughness of the surface of the skin, which is associated with itching, scaling and dryness. Sometimes fish-like scales may also shed off. It may be black or red in color; usually the periphery is red and occasionally there may be oozing of yellowish fluid. All these conditions develop accordingly to the pathogenic substances.

Qooba is a roughness which appears over the surface of the skin in which the skin becomes peeled and scales shed off. Initially, it appears as a small spot over the skin surface which spread peripherally to acquire a large surface area in an annular fashion.

It resembles Sa'afa, especially sa'afa-e-yabisa. It may be huzaz but according to some, huzaz is the Qooba of the scalp.

It is a type of roughness on the skin in the form of a circular hyper-pigmented patch having edges. It is associated with itching but is devoid of pain.

QOOBA (DERMATOPHYTOSIS)

HISTORY REVIEW

Qooba is one of the oldest and commonest, skin disease existing even before its true mycological nature was established.

The first recorded reference to a dermatophyte infection is attributed to **Aulus Cornelium Celsus,** the Roman encyclopaedist, who, in the treatise De Re Medicina, written around 30 A.D, described a suppurative infection of the scalp that came to be known as the Kerion of Celsus. In this era and down through the Middle Ages, the various Dermatophytosis were described as tinea.

Dioscorides, in **60 A.D.,** gave the description of Qooba in children and its treatment in De Materia Medica.

Jalinoos (Galen 129-200 A.D.), described Qooba, its cause and treatment and classified it into acute and chronic in his book Mayameer.

Rabban Tabri (810-895 A.D), in his book Firdausul Hikmat, has made a mention of Qooba, its causes and treatment based on humoral theory. He classified Qooba into three types, viz: Qooba damvi- which occurs due to fasad and ratubat-e-fasida, Qooba ratubi- which occurs due to fasid-e-ratubat and ufunat (infection) and Qooba saudavi- which occurs due to khilt-e-sauda.

Zakariya Razi (850-923 A.D), the author of Al Havi fit-Tib, described Qooba quiet broadly and classified into Qooba ratab and Qooba yabis. Besides, he also gave various

5

regimes for its treatment. He also mentioned that application of oil is beneficial in the treatment of Qooba.

Hasan Al-Qamari (9th Century A.D), quoted in Ghina Muna that Qooba is caused by sanguine humour which is burnt and converted into morbid melancholic humour.

Ali Ibn Abbas Majoosi (930-999 A.D.), in this book Kamil-us-Sana'a discussed Qooba, its causes, clinical presentation and treatment.

Ibn-e-Sina (980-1037 A.D), the author of Canon of Medicine, extensively described Qooba and classified it according to its causes, clinical presentation and mentioned that it is seasonal disease which appears in fasl-e-Kharif i.e. the rainy season. According to him, Qooba and Daad are synonyms. He found no difference between Qooba and sa'afa either. Following the humoral basis, he considered it to be primarily a melancholic disorder but added that some of its types may be sanguineous and phlegmatic too.

Ahmad Al-Tabri (10th Century A.D), has given a comprehensive description of the disease in his famous book 'Al-Moalijat-e-Buqratiya'. He stated that the disease is similar to shara (urticaria) which affects the skin surface. Regarding the etiopathogenesis of the disease, he stated that irritating pathogenic matter or substance escapes out of capillaries, resulting in the formation of hyperpigmented spot/papule, which later spreads and takes large rounded/circular patch.

Ismail Jurjani (12th Century A.D), in "Zakheera Khawazam Shahi", an encyclopedia of medicine, described Qooba in detail. It is known as paryun in Persian. He mentioned two causes for its occurrence, which are Khilt-e-bad (noxious humour) and Quwat-e-tabiyat (corrective faculty).

Akbar Arzani (17th Century A.D.), considered Qooba as a roughness over the skin surface which is devoid of pain but associated with itching, redness, and hyperpigmentation.

Daud Antaki (1514-1599 A.D) differentiated Qooba from huzaz (kerion in scalp). According to him, the consumption of certain food items like meat of camel and weak buffalo can be blamed for development of Qooba.

Azam Khan (19th Century A.D), explained Qooba as a roughness over the skin associated with itching and scaling and red periphery. He also discussed its prognosis and complications. According to him, it occurs due to the deranged blood in which mirra sauda is mixed and sometimes due to balgham-e-borqi which takes the chronic form of Qooba. In chronic conditions, scales like that of fish are formed. Similar scales are found in sa'afa-e-yabisa.

Raymond Sabouraud classified the dermatophytes into four genera, viz: Achorion, Epidermophyton, Microsporum and Trichophyton primarily on the basis of the clinical aspects of the disease, combined with cultural and microscopic observations. The medium that he developed is still used today for culturing fungi (although the ingredients are modified) and is named Sabouraud Dextrose Agar (SDA) after him. In the meantime, wood's lamp was invested by the Baltimore physicist, Robert W. Wood that was used for detection of fungal infection of hair in 1925.

Chester Emmons, in 1934, critically reviewed the taxonomic status of the dermatophytes and recognized only three genera-Microsporum, Trichophyton and Epidermophyton on the basis of mycological principles.

EPIDEMIOLOGY

In general, Dermatophytosis has a prevalence of around 20-25% throughout the world.[158] Over USD 500,000,000 per year is spent worldwide for drugs targeted against dermatophytoses.[35] T. rubrum is found to be the most common dermatophyte for tinea corporis, tinea cruris, tinea pedis and tinea unguium worldwide.

Foster et al. published a detailed survey from 1999-2002, in which T. rubrum remained the most prevalent pathogen, and an increased incidence of this dermatophyte was observed in finger and toe nails, i.e., onychomycosis (from 64.4% to 79.3%), as well as tinea corporis and cruris (from 32% to 47%), T. manuum (from 64.4 to 80%), and T. pedis (from 56.8% to 82.9%). However, the incidence of T. tonsurans in tinea capitis increased continuously (from 89.3% to 95.8%). The Africans, the Americans and the Hispanics have a higher incidence of T. capitis.

In Japan, skin disease caused by geophilic fungi is decreasing while case reports of zoonoses from various animals are increasing. Tinea pedis is the commonest dermatophyte infections in Japan. T. rubrum is presumed to be the dominant pathogen of this disease. In the United Kingdom, in the late 1950s, the Zoophilic dermatophytes M.canis, T.verrucosum, were the two most prevalent dermatophytes infecting the scalp.

QOOBA (DERMATOPHYTOSIS)

In India, superficial infection of the skin nails and hair accounts for 8-10% of all skin outpatient attendance. Tinea cruris and corporis are the commonest varieties seen in India, followed by Tinea pedis, captitis, barbae, unguium and manuum in descending order of frequency. Etiologically, T. rubrum tops the list followed by T. mentagrophyte and E. floccosum, T. verrrucosum, M. canis and M. gypseum.

ETIOLOGY

A. UNANI CONCEPT

According to the Unani system of medicine, the concept of four humours (Akhlat-e-Arba'a) forms the basis of health and disease. The derangement in the equilibrium of these humours results in Qooba, as described in various classical texts.

Ismail Jurjani has broadly classified its causes into two.

- Khilt-e-bad: Which may further be classified into two types:

  Khilt-e-tez and raqeeq: Produces lesions which are moist and have a burning sensation.

  Khilt-e-ghaleez and saudavi: Lesions are dry and burning sensation is less.

- Quwat-e-tabiyat (corrective faculty): It is also responsible for Qooba as it diverts khilt-e-bad/ khilt-e-rabbi (noxious humour) from vital organs towards the skin surface, rendering them safe. Hence, any alteration in the corrective faculty may predispose to Qooba.

The cause of Qooba is similar to that of the sa'afa; that is, the haad (sharp), harrif (astringent) or pungent fluid is mixed with ghaleez saudavi maadda (viscous melancholic humour) and is more viscid than the matter of jarb (scabies). And it may also occur due to balgham-e-maleh (saline phlegm), which is burnt and converted into sauda (melancholic humour).

Qooba is caused by fasad-e-dam (morbid blood) due to viscous matters. If the matter is hot and has less fluid that there will be dry Qooba.

Qooba may develop due to acute liquefied fluid of blood, mixed with black bile. And it may be due to melancholic humour, i.e., black bile.

The dry Qooba occur due to melancholic humour and the moist one due to melancholic humour mixed with blood. It may be due to the mixture of latif khun and mirra sauda (abnormal black bile) and sometimes due to the admixture of ghaliz ratubat (viscid substances) with balgham-e-shor (abnormal phlegm). Ufunat is also one of the causes of Qooba as quoted in Aksir-e-Azam.

B. MODERN CONCEPT

According to modern medicine, the sole cause of Dermatophytosis is dermatophytes.

Dermatophytes:

Dermatophytes have been defined as keratinophilic organisms that have the ability to invade the hair, nails, and the skin of the living host.

QOOBA (DERMATOPHYTOSIS)

Taxonomical classification of dermatophytes

Kingdom-Fungi

Phylum- Ascomycota/Dikaryamycota

Order- Onygenales

Class- Arthroderma, Nannizia

Genus-Microsporum, Trichophyton, Epidermophyton

On the basis of morphology, dermatophytes and classified into 3 genera:

- **Trichophyton:** This genus contains 22 species. The important ones are T. rubrum, T. mentagrophyte and T. violaceum. This genus includes both human and animal species. It affects the hair, the glabrous skin, and the nails. They are ectothrix as well as endothix fungi. It also produces macro and micro conidia. Macroconidia vary in morphology. They may appear cylindrical or club-shaped. They are smooth surfaced, thin-walled and may have elongated ends. They measure 20-50 X 4-6 um with upto 8 septa.

- **Microsporum:** This genus contains 17 species, the important ones being M. audounii (human variety) and M. canis (animal variety). They mainly affect the hair and less commonly the glabrous skin. They are ectothix fungi. Nails are usually not affected. This genus produces macroconidia as well as microconidia but the former are predominant. Macroconidia are spindle shaped with slightly tapering ends, symmetrical, rough-surfaced and thick-walled. They may be very large, measuring 40-120 X 7-30 um with up to 16 septa.

- **Epidermophyton:** This genus has two known species, of which only E. floccosum is pathogenic. It affects the human skin and the nails, sparing the hair.[56] The genus is characterized by large macroconidia which are oval or club-shaped and clustered in branches, smooth, thin-to-moderately-thick walled with 1-9 septa. They measure 20-60 X 4-13um with upto 9 septa.

Ecological classification

There are three ecological groups of dermatophytes according to their natural habitat.

- **Zoophilic:** They are basically animal pathogens, but occasionally infect humans. Domestic animals and pets are becoming and increasing source of these infections in urban areas. They can be transmitted to humans sporadically. Transmission can occur through direct contact with the infected animal or indirectly through inanimate objects. Infections caused by zoophilic organisms are inflammatory and short lasting in humans. Examples are T.verrucosum and M. Canis.

- **Geophilic:** The strains cultured from humans are found to be more virulent and are responsible for epidemics of the disease under favorable conditions. Infections caused by them are also inflammatory and seen sporadically in humans. The commonest geophile isolated in human infections is M. gypseum.

- **Anthropophilic:** They are associated primarily with human and rarely infect animals. They are transmitted from one person to another by direct contact or indirectly through fomites. They usually produce mild but chronic infections. The lesions may be inflammatory or non-inflammatory. Examples are T. rubrum, M. audouinii and E. floccosum.

Table 1: Ecology of Common Human Dermatophyte Species.

Species	Natural Habitat	Incidence
Epidermophyton floccosum	Humans	Common
Trichophyton rubrum	Humans	Very Common
Trichophyton interdigitale	Humans	Very Common
Trichophyton tonsurans	Humans	Common
Trichophyton violaceum	Humans	Less Common
Trichophyton concentricum	Humans	Rare*
Trichophyton schoenleinii	Humans	Rare*
Trichophyton soudanense	Humans	Rare*
Microsporum audouinii	Humans	Less Common*
Microsporum ferrugineum	Humans	Less Common*
Trichophyton mentagrophytes	Mice, rodents	Common
Trichophyton equinum	Horses	Rare
Trichophyton erinacei	Hedgehogs	Rare*
Trichophyton verrucosum	Cattle	Rare
Microsporum canis	Cats	Common
Microsporum gypseum	Soil	Common
Microsporum nanum	Soil/Pigs	Rare
Microsporum cookie	Soil	Rare

- *Geographically restricted

- Das JK, Sengupta S, Gangopadhyay A. Dermatophyte infection of the male genitalia. Indian J Dermatol;2009; 54:21-3

Host Factors

- **Age:** Prepubertal children between 6 months and 12 years, especially boys, are more susceptible to tinea capitis. The adults are spared from T. capitis because of the presence of sebum, which is absent in prepubertal children.

- **Sex:** Dermatophyte infections are, in general, more common in males. T. capitis is more common in boys than girls. This is due to the shortness of hair in boys and the ease with which the spores can reach the scalp. T. cruris is more prevalent in males, the M:F is 2.5:1 to 3:1.7. T. barbae is seen only in males.

- **Socioeconomic Status:** It commonly occurs under poor hygienic conditions. Its prevalence remains low in developed countries. Athlete's foot or T. pedis, the most widely suffered dermatophyte infection, is considered a disease of affluence and high standard of living due to more use of occlusive footwear.

- **Customs and Habits:** Vegetable oils were believed to be a protective factor against acquiring T. capitis. Mustard oil used in North and North east India for hair dressing was found to have an inhibitory effect on fungi affecting the scalp, People who use occlusive footwear have an increased incidence of T. pedis. Some other contributing factors include indigestion, and wearing of dirty and moist clothes.

- **Associated diseases:** Susceptibility to persistent dermatophyte infection has been associated with a number of underlying conditions such as diabetes mellitus, Cushing's syndrome and Lymphoma, frequent usage of antibiotics, immunosuppressive drugs, and organ transplantation. Familial endocrinopathies and condition of defective CMI responses like collagen vascular diseases alter the clinical appearance and course of infection. Staphylococcus aureus infection enhances the degree of inflammation in dermatophytosis.

- **Endocrine and Metabolic Factors:** Hormonal factors may predispose to infection; the female hormone progesterone is an effective inhibitor of fungal growth. Therefore, females are more likely to skip the infections. The male dihydrotestosterone is an effective inhibitor of progesterone binding site. So males are at more risk of developing Dermatophytosis.

- **Dietary Factors:** Deficiency of proteins and vitamin A is the predisposing factor, especially for T. capitis. The consumption of camel and weak buffalo meat and excessive sweets is thought to be the contributing factor. Excessive consumption of sweetened food items also predisposes to the development of Qooba.

- **Environmental Factors:** It is a disease of fasl-e-kharif (rainy season). Majorities of the cases of Dermatophytosis are seen during the rainy season. The frequency of fungal infection varies with seasons. The highest number of tinea pedis and cruris occurred in summer, while tinea capitis, corporis, and unguium occurred in spring and winter months.

PATHOGENESIS

Tabiyat (Natural Power) is the driving force which pulls out the morbid matters from Aaza-e-Raeesa (Principal Organs) and expels them towards the surface of the skin. This morbid matter is composed of Akhlat-e-Harra wa Lateefa (hot and thin humours) mixed with Akhlat-e-Arzia wa Ghaleeza (thick and early Humours). Due to this duplicity in the nature of Akhlat, the disease spreads in both directions. It spreads rapidly due to the Hiddat (acuteness) and Latafat (thinness) of the Maadda (Matter), while the spread is slow owing to the thickness and tardiness of the Maadda. Moreover, the disease both fulminates and heals faster if there is preponderance of Akhlat-e-Harra in the causative material, while it develops and heals slowly if Akhlat-e-Arzia are in excess.

The invasion of the epidermis by dermatophytes follows a common pattern, starting with adherence between arthroconidia and keratinocytes, followed by penetration through and between cells and the development of host response. Some investigators have found that dermatophytes prefer to spread between horn cells of the stratum corneum rather than through them, as might be postulated in a keratin digestion process. It is difficult for the fungi to invade the normal or the intact skin surface. Hence, the presence of suitable environment on the host skin is of utmost importance in the development of clinical dermatophytosis. The factors that favor the inoculation of fungi in the skin surface are trauma, maceration and increased hydration of the skin. Different species of Dermatophytosis are attracted to different types of keratins, e.g. T. rubrum seldom affects the hair but frequently involves the nails and glabrous skin, whereas E. floccosum rarely involves the nails and never affects the hair. These variations are presumably due to differences in the type of keratin or in the ability of the organism to organism to metabolize this material.

A. Skin: Kligman, divided the pathogenesis of the disease into the following stages:

- **Period of incubation** - During this stage the dematophyte grows into the stratum corneum, and sometimes with minimal clinical signs.

- **Period of enlargement** – The lesion becomes clinically evident and it enlarges at this stage. The size and the duration of the lesion in the stratum corneum are determined by the rate of growth of organisms and the epidermal turnover rate. The fungal growth rate must equal or exceed the epidermal turnover rate. Labeling indices reveal that in an annular dermatophytic lesion there is a four-fold increase in the epidermal turnover at the inflammatory periphery of the lesion, while in other areas of the lesion it is comparable to that of normal skin. It appears that the inflammatory responses at the periphery of the lesion stimulates an increased epidermal turnover in an effort to shed the organisms. As the lesion advances peripherally, it leaves a central area of clearing. This newly healed skin of the central area of the lesion is usually resistant to further infection. Sometimes the central clearing is incomplete due to very little inflammation, which is not enough to eliminate the fungus. It may also be due to lowered turnover rate which in turn is influenced by the degree of inflammation. Such a condition gives rise to chronic infection. Central clearance is often partial in tinea imbricate due to T.

concentricum, in which successive ways of fungal growth occurs in the skin previously cleared of infection, but overall mycelial expansion is centrifugal.

- **Refractory period** – The fungus ceases to grow after the clinical lesion has attained a particular size.
- **Stage of involution** – In this stage there is a decrease in signs and symptoms.

A carrier stage may also be found when the presence of dermatophyte is detected in apparently normal skin by KOH examination or culture.

B. Hairs: The pathogenesis of tinea capitis has been studied by Kligman and by Freedman and Howard. From the classical experimental work of Kligman on Microsporum audouinii, it is evident that invasion of stratum corneum of the scalp skin is an absolute necessity to cause actual hair infection. Minor trauma assists inoculation, which is followed, after approximately 3 weeks, by clinical evidence of hair shaft infection. After the invasion of the perifollicular stratum corneum, the fungi invade the hair follicle at the mid follicular level from the adjacent stratum corneum. The hyphae descend within the intra-pilary portion of hair until they reach the border of the keratogenous zone. The terminal tuft of hyphae in this location is termed **Adamson's fringe.** The infected hair, when plucked breaks at its weakest point which is just above Adamson's fringe.

C. Nails: Onychomycosis commonly begins from the lateral ends of free nail plate distally and then involves the nail bed and subsequently the nail plate. Involvement of the nail bed leads to the deposition of a powdery material under the distal portion of the nail plate while involvement of the nail plate may lead to its thickening, with discoloration and a dull surface. If the nail plate becomes brittle, it produces the appearance as if the nail plate has been eaten-up. Subungual hyperkeratosis results from a hyper-proliferative reaction of the nail bed in response to the infection. Gradually, the entire portion becomes brittle and separates from its nail bed as a result of piling up of subungual keratin (debris).

IMMUNOLOGY

Various reviews on immune mechanism regarding Dermatophytosis have been explained, but the excellent ones have been written by Weitzman and Summerbill. Wagner and Sohnle, Jones, Dahl, Emmons et al., and Ahmad. Resistance or natural defense against dermatophyte infections may involve nonimmunologic as well as immunologic mechanisms. Natural resistance in cases of T. capitis may be conferred by increase in fungistatic and fungicidal long chain fatty acids, which occur after puberty. the $\alpha2$ macroglobulin and keratinase inhibitor modifies the growth of organisms. Transferin binds to irons that dermatophytes need for continuous growth. Serum inhibitory factor(SIF), probably an unsaturated tranferin, appears to limit the growth of the dermatophytes to the stratum corneum under most circumstances. Dermatophytes elicit both humoral and cell mediated immunity (CMI). But he major immunologic defense mechanism is type IV hypersensitivity response, while the humoral limb of the immune system plays a minor role in the development of acquired resistance against dermatophytes. Two major classes of antigens, the glycopeptides and the keratinases, mainly contribute to the immune mechanism. The protein portion of the glycopeptides preferentially stimulates the CMI while its polysaccharide portion preferentially stimulates the humoral immunity. The keratinases produces by the dermatophytes aid them to penetrate in the skin easily. They also elicit delayed type hypersensitivity (DTH) responses when injected intradermally into the skin of experimental animals. If the individual has previously never been exposed to the fungus in question, it is noted by the lymphocytes, leading to a cellular immune reaction, usually in about a week or so. Jones and coworkers showed that delayed-type hypersensitivity developed at that time. Lymphocyte transformation studies become positive as the skin test becomes positive.

HISTOPATHOLOGY

Ackerman has described three distinct histological changes produced by dermatophytes in the infected tissue. These changes are: the presence of neutrophils, compact orthokeratosis, and the presence of sandwich sign. The sandwich sign refers to fungal elements sandwiched between the normal orthokeratosis at the surface of the skin and altered keratin beneath it. The epidermis is often spongiotic and more florid spongiotic vesiculation is usually present when the palms and soles are involved. The dermis shows mild superficial oedema and the sparse perivascular infiltrate, which includes lymphocytes and occasionally eosinophils or neutrophils.

CLINICAL PRESENTATION AND CLASSIFICATION

UNANI CONCEPT

The clinical presentation and classification of the disease have been described according to their causative substances in various Unani classical texts by various physicians and writers of Unani system of medicine.

Zakaria Razi has classified it into two types:

- **Damvi (Ratab):** It present as a reddish discoloration associated with oozing on itching. It is produced by dam (blood), burnt and converted into sauda (black bile). It disappears easily on treatment.
- **Saudavi (Yabis):** It presents as a whitish discoloration. This is produced by balgham that becomes hot and saline and converts into sauda.

Ibne Sina classified it accordingly to the cause, disease pattern and appearance.

- **Damvi (Ratab):** There will be oozing in this type, but it is easily curable.
- **Saudavi (Yabis):** It is produced by sauda, which is formed by the ihteraq (combustion) of balgham-e-maleh (saline phlegm).
- **Mutaqashshir:** It is characterized by scaling due to extreme dryness. It may be deep seated sometimes and resembles bars-e-aswad, or it may appear like slough.
- **Ghair mutaqashshir:** It does not scale.
- **Saee Khabees:** It is spreading in nature and not easily curable.
- **Waqif:** It is localized and does not spread.

- **Haad:** It is of short duration, acute in condition, but easily curable.

- **Raddi:** It has poor prognosis and is not easily curable.

Qooba appears as a roughness and desquamation over the skin surface in which scales shed off from the skin. It seems to be bars-e-aswad that did not reach up to that extent of disease.

Qooba clinically presents accordingly to its causative humours. It appears as a roughness which is associated with itching. There will be oozing of fluid if the cause is khilt-e-ratab, and scaling is associated with khilt-e-yabis.

Qooba is characterized by itching and burning. The oozing of fluid is also present, if the cause is khilt-e-raqeeq haad. In case of ghaleez khilt-e-sauda, there will be more dryness and roughness in the skin, and lesser itching and burning than in khilt-e-raqeeq. There may be common presentation of features of both the types, if the cause is mixed with both.

Rabban Tabri has given a more detailed account of clinical features of Qooba. He has quoted that Qooba resembles shara (urticaria) which spreads over the skin surface. Initially, it appears as a small lesion or a dot like spot, which advances circumferentially, and acquires a large area by spreading over the skin surface. This presentation appears particularly over a superficial skin.

Rabban Tabri has broadly classified Qooba into three type:

- **Damvi:** It is produced by khilt-e-dam or ratubat-e-fasidah (morbid fluids).

- **Ratubi:** It appears due to fasad-e-ratubat and ufunat (infection)
- **Saudavi:** Produced by akhlat that gets burnt and is converted into sauda.

Apart from the above mentioned types he also maintains that, every now and then, Qooba produces painful condition due to the involvement of safra that produces hiddat in the causative matter. But the patient feels a pleasant sensation in the case where khilt-e-hareef (pungent humour) is involved.

On the basis of the depth of involvement, two types of Qooba have been mentioned in Ghina Muna.

- **Kaghzi daad:** When the disease is superficial.
- **Bhainsya daad:** When the invasion is up to the sub-cutaneous tissue.

Qooba appears as a roughness on the skin surface and is associated with itching. It is either reddish or blackish; usually the periphery and the centre are red. The disease is either localized or generalized, or it may be acute or chronic, in which scales shed off from the skin. Sometimes oozing of yellow fluid is also associated with the disease. Qooba resembles sa'afa-e-yabis. Another different type is Qooba Khabees (malignant) that predisposes to juzam (leprosy). All these conditions develop due to the hiddat, khabasat, latafat, and kasafat of the causative matters. A different entity of Qooba is jarabia, in which itching predominates and commonly involves the area of the skin over the scrotum.[95] Akuta is a type of Qooba found on the back and dorsum of hands.

MODERN CLASSIFICATION

The clinical features of dermatophyte infections result from a combination of keratin destruction and as inflammatory host response. A typical lesion of Dermatophytosis is an annular scaling patch with raised margin showing a variable degree of inflammation, the center usually being less inflamed than the edge. The wide variation in clinical presentation depends upon the species and probably the strain of the fungus concerned, size of inoculum, and site of the body infected and immune status of the host.

1. TINEA CORPORIS

Synonyms: Tinea circinata or Tinea glabrosa, Ringworm of body.

It is the dermatophyte infection of the glabrous skin, with the exclusion of certain specific regions (i.e., hands feet groin and face). All the species belonging to the three genera of dermatophytes can cause Tinea corporis. The three most common causative organisms are T. rubrum, M. canis and T. mentagrophytes. The infection is more common in adult males. Children appear to have an increased incidence of tinea corporis caused by zoophilic organisms.

The characteristic presentation is an annular lesion with an active erythematous and sometimes vesicular border. As the lesion progresses, central clearing occurs. The degree of inflammation varies depending on the species of the fungus, the host's immune response and the extent of follicular invasion. Pustules and vesicles are abundant in predominantly inflammatory lesions, while scaling is the most prominent finding in less inflammatory lesions. Not all cases of tinea corporis reveal the characteristic features described above. Central clearing may be lacking. The central skin may show post inflammatory pigmentation, a change of texture or residual erythematous dermal nodules. Scaling of the active border may be almost absent, and redness may be minimal. Infections with T. rubrum can take this aspect with very chronic, non-inflammatory, extensive lesions.

Types of Tinea Corporis

- **Tinea Imbricata (Tokelau):** It is also known as "tinea circinata tropical". The name imbricate is derived from imbrex meaning shingle. Shingle also refers to herpes zoster and it means tiled. The infection is probably contracted in childhood and can persist for lifetime. There is some evidence that susceptibility to tinea imbricatta is determined hereditarily through an autosomal recessive trait. The causative organism is the anthropophilic T. concentricum. The fully developed skin lesion is characteristically polycyclic, concentric and has lamellar plaques of scales with slight erythema, scattered throughout the body, resembling "erythema gyratum repens". Itching is present only at the outset. Central clearance is often partial in T. imbricatta.

- **Tinea Corporis Gladiatorum:** It is clinical variant T. corporis that occurs among competitive wrestlers: most out-breaks are caused by T. tonsurans by person to person contact. Characteristic lesions have a rough scaly circular border with central clearing. They may vary from small to large patches.

- **Tinea Incognito:** It was first described by Ive and Marks in the year 1968. It refers to a dermatophyte infection that has been modified clinically by the use of corticosteroids, either systemic or topical. As most of the patients are generally immunosuppressed, the annular scaling and the circumscribed borders are absent, leading to a diffuse erythema with follicular papules and pustules. It occurs due to intrafollicular invasion by the fungus. Kerion like lesions and dermal nodules may be present.

- **Majocchi's Granuloma:** It is also known as Granuloma tricofitico, granuloma trichophyticum and nodular granulomatous perifolliculitis. It was, for the first time, described by Majocchi Dmenico in the year 1883. Earlier T. violaceum was the most common etiologic agent, but now it is T. rubrum. It occurs when dermatophytes gain access to the deeper layers of the skin up to the reticular dermis, which is not the case in usual setting. Clinically, it is characterized by nonpruritic solitary or multiple persistent papulopustules, plaques or oval patches. They may be scaly. Majocchi's granuloma is of further two types: the follicular type and the subcutaneous nodular type. The former, occurs mainly due to trauma and is commonly seen in women who repeatedly shave their legs. In men, prolonged maceration from boots may play a role. The subcutaneous nodular type occurs in immunocompromised individuals.

- **Agminate folliculitis:** It is caused by zoophilic organisms. Clinically it is characterized by well defined erythematous plaques studded with perifollicular pustules.

2. TINEA CRURIS

Synonyms: Dhobi itch, Jock Itch, Crotch itch, Eczema marginatum.

It is a dermatophyte infection of the groin. It includes infection of the genitalia, pubic area and perineal area, occasionally the upper thighs. The Predominant cause is anthropophilic species, T. rubrum most commonly, but T. interdigitale is also not rare. In addition, E. floccosum is now rarely involved. However, in the previous century, this dermatophyte species was a very common agent of the disease, and it was even known with the name of E. inguinale.

The disease is worldwide in distribution, but it is found more commonly in hot climates. Warm and humid climate as in India, particularly the monsoon season, favors tinea cruris. Also tight-fitting, sweaty or rubbing clothing or undergarments are the favoring factor.

The lesions are usually bilateral but asymmetrical. They begin on the inguinal creases and take a semicircular aspect. Lesions caused by E. floccosum seldom extend beyond the genitocrural fold and medial upper thing. But the lesions caused by T. rubrum extend both distally on the medial part of the thighs, and proximally to the lower abdomen and pubic area, the perineum and buttocks. The peripheral activity is characterized by fine scaling and the presence of some papules, vesicles and pustules. The borders are sharply demarcated. Scaling is variable and, occasionally, may mask the inflammatory changes. In the more acute forms, the lesions may be moist and exudative or can have an eczematous aspect (historical name: eczema marginatum hebra). In the chronic form, the lesions are dry and annular. T. cruris causes itching or a burning sensation and rubbing and scratching, lichenification or impetiginisation can complicate the condition. It rarely involves the scrotum or labia majora. This contrasts with the case of inguinal candidiasis.

3. TINEA FACIEI

Synonyms: Tinea faciale.

It is the dermatophyte infection of the face, apart from beard and moustache area. Also, by definition, all dermatophyte infections of the face in women and prepubertal boys are tinea faciei.[54] It is commonly caused by T. rubrum and T. mentagrophytes and occasionally by M. audounii and M. canis.

Tinea faciale usually presents as erythematous, slightly scaling, pruritic lesion with indistinct brothers. It is associated with photosensitivity. Atypical features are more common in T. faciei than in other forms of dermatophytosis. Neonatal cases, though rare, have also been reported.

4. TINEA CAPITIS

Synonyms: Tinea tonsurans.

It is Dermatophytosis of the scalp and the associated hair and hair follicle. It can be caused by all pathogenic dermatophytes except for E. floccosum, and T. rubrum. The disease commonly affects children, boys much more often than girls. It may develop as a consequence of shared headgear, e.g., comb or hairbrush.

There are four clinical patterns of Tinea capitis:

- **Seborrheic Pattern/ Grey patch/ Non-inflammatory/ Human or epidemic type:** The infection closely resembles seborrheic dermatitis. Lesions are usually asymptomatic. Some patients complain of mild itching. It is characterized by one or more well demarcated patches, often circular in shape, with dandruff like scaling usually on the occiput. Hair in the infected area is grey and lusterless due to coating of arthroconidia and hence the name grey patch is often used. Hair frequently breaks off just above the level of the scalp, rather than being shedding entirely.

- **Black dot Pattern:** The endothix infection causes the hair shaft to weaken and break off at the level of the scalp, leaving a black dot on the scalp. This pattern is primarily associated with the T. tonsurans or T. violaceum infection. When the hair loss occurs, the affected areas are characteristically multiple and polygonal in outline, with distinct finger-like margins. The lesions may occasionally be inflammatory, ranging from pustular folliculitis to furuncle-like lesions or obvious kerions. In some instances the lesions may appear without obvious black dots.

- **Kerion Pattern/ inflammatory type:** Kerion was first described by Celsus in the first century A.D.[25] In most cases this violent reaction results from zoophilic T. verrucosum or T. mentagrophytes. It is a painful inflammatory, boggy, indurated, tender mass, studded with broken or unbroken hair, vesicles and pustules. There is oozing of purulent material from follicular orificies. Thick crusting with matting of adjacent hair is common. The patient usually has posterior cervical lymphadenopathy. Secondary bacterial infection may further aggravate the condition. It may heal with scarring, resulting in permanent alopecia. Id reaction frequently occurs in the form of lichenoid papules running down from scalp to trunk. Erythema nodosum may also occur in association.

- **Favus Pattern/ Tinea favosa:** Favus is a Latin word which refers to a honeycomb appearance. Favus is now rare and occurs due to T. schoenleinii and occasionally due to T. violaceum or M. gypsum. It is also an inflammatory type of tinea capitis which begins early in life and commonly extends into adulthood. The infection is characterized by the formation of scutulae and a chronic evolution, ending in many cases, in scarring alopecia. The term scutulae refer to the shield shape. It appears as a yellow cup-shaped crust with concavity facing upwards and is pierced by hair. Adjacent crusts enlarge to become confluent and form a yellow crusting mass. The borders of the lesions are often polycyclic. A characteristic mousy odor may be observed.

5. TINEA BARBAE

Synonyms: Tinea sycosis and Barber's Itch.

It is the dermatophyte infection limited to the bread and moustache area with invasion of coarse hair. It is seen in adult males. It is more common in rural settings, often affecting dairy farmers and cattle ranchers. In most cases, the zoophilic ectothrix fungi T. verrucosum and T. mentagrophytes are responsible for this type of infection. M. canis is a less common cause. Usually the infection is contracted by exposure to animals. Transmission from person to person is via contaminated barber's razors or clippers.

QOOBA (DERMATOPHYTOSIS)

Tinea barbae may be of the following types:

- **Inflammatory or Kerion-Like or deep type:** Most often caused by T. mentagrophytes and T. verrucosum, this variety is analogous to the kerion formation in tinea capitis. The lesions are usually unilateral. They are commonly seen on the chin, neck and maxillary or sub maxillary areas. There is sparing of the upper lip area. The lesions are nodular and boggy and there is often an associated weeping of seropurulent material with subsequent crusting. Perifollicular pustules are also seen. Coalescence of these inflammatory areas yields abscess like collection of pus. The overlying skin s inflamed. The hair is loose and gets easily plucked. Scarring and permanent alopecia may eventually occur in severely inflamed individuals.

- **Superficial or Sycosiform Type**: The causative organisms are the relatively non-inflammatory anthropophiles (T. violaceum and T. rubrum) In this type of tinea barbae there is diffuse erythema with perifollicular papules and pustules that resemble bacterial follliculitis. Hair invasion depends upon the organism involved, e.g., T. violaceum infection results in brittle, lusterless hair due to endothrix infection. Conversely, T. rubrum infections produce hair invasion less often. When the hair is extracted the bulb appears intact.

- **Circinate or Spreading Type**: This variant presents with lesions similar to those found in tinea circinata of glabrous skin, with an active, spreading vesiculopustular border and central scaling. There may be relative sparing of hair in this variant.

- **Atypical Lesions:** The lesions of tinea barbae may present in an atypical manner, especially if the disease is altered by glucocorticoides or other therapy. They may be granuloma annular-like or abscess-like tumours with M. canis, and verrucous granulomatous lesions with E. floccosum (verrucous epidermophyton).

6. TINEA MANUUM

Tinea Manuum is the dermatophyte infection of the palmer and the interdigital area of the hand. It is commonly caused by T. rubrum and E. floccosum, and in most cases, there is a pre-existing foot infection, with or without nail involvement (two feet-- one-hand-syndrome) particularly in t. rubrum infections.

The infection is usually unilateral, the right hand being more commonly affected than the left. The lesion on the dorsum appears similar to those of tinea corporis. There are 2 types of tinea manuum:

- **Non-inflammatory or squamous type:** It is the commoner clinical presentation of tinea manuum. It presents as a mild asymptomatic scaling to diffuse scaling hyperkeratosis. Accentuation of palmer creases is a characteristic feature. Hyperhydrosis is commonly associated with this type of tinea manuum.
- **Inflammatory vesicular/ dyshydrotic/ eczematous type:** Vesicles, usually multiloculated, occur in clusters principally on the palms but rarely on the dorsal surface. If the diseased hand is not subjected to constant chemical or traumatic irritation, the lesion heals spontaneously. Bullous tinea manuum, described

recently, is caused by T. verrucosum. In addition to the factors described above, repeated trauma and topical steroids may cause bullous lesions.

7. TINEA PEDIS

Synonyms: Athlete's foot.

Tinea pedis is the Dermatophytosis of the plantar surface, interdigital and subdigital areas. The main organism involved is the anthropophilic species T. rubrum and, less commonly, T. mentagrophytes var interdigitale and E. floccosum. The usual agent is, however, T. rubrum, but non-dermatophytes such as Hendersonula toruloidea or Syntalidium hyalinium can also produce a similar picture. T. rubrum is often associated with chronic, non-inflammatory, erythematosquamous reactions. Infections due to T. mentagrophytes var. interdigitale often lead to vesicular or bullous inflammatory lesions. E. floccosum may produce both types of reactions, but infect toenails less significantly. Tinea pedis is the commonest form of dermatophyte infection in developed countries. The interdigital type is the most common subtype. It is more common in adolescents but rare in pre pubertal children. The infection rate is higher with the use of community baths or pools. Cultures from swimming pool or washroom floors as well as items of clothing in contact with infected areas are positive for the responsible organism. The infection may be less prevalent in societies that do not commonly wear shoes. Therefore, in India it is comparatively less common due to the habit of going barefoot or wearing open sandals. Patients with a history of atopic dermatitis have an increased incidence of tinea pedis.

Tinea pedis is reported to be relatively frequent in patients with hereditary palmoplanter keratosis.

The individual may exhibit 'two feet one hand' pattern, where the development of tinea pedis precedes the development of tinea manuum.

The clinical manifestations of the infection are altered in patients with T-lymphocyte abnormalities, including those with acquired immunodeficiency syndrome (AIDS), in whom there is often an extensive spread of the lesion on to the dorsal surface of the foot.

There are four clinical types of Tinea pedis:

- **Chronic Interdigital Tinea Pedis:** It is most common clinical form, commonly referred to as 'athlete's foot'. It is dermatophyte infection involving the web spaces of the feet. Some or all web spaces are involved, with the space between the fourth and fifth toes most commonly affected. The clinical presentation may be characterized by dryness, scaling and fissuring or by white, moist maceration. Irritation and itching are often present (simplex type). The symptomatic picture of athlete's foot results from the interaction of bacteria as well as dermatophytes. The presence of dermatophytes alone or overgrowth of bacteria alone produces a relatively mild picture that is short-lived and relatively asymptomatic.

- **Chronic papulosquamous Tinea Pedis (Moccasin Type):** In the mildest form, a few small scaly collarettes can be found. In more severe forms, diffuse, dry slivery white scaly lesions, covering a mild pink to red inflamed skin, are present. In the most severe cases, the soles, heels and sides of the feet are affected. The patients complain of a dry, scaly skin, resistant to emollients. This type is also known as "moccasin foot". It is usually bilateral, involvement of the dorsum of the foot is rare, but onychomycosis is common.

- **Vesicular or vesicobullous type of Tinea Pedis (Dyshidrosis Type):** A vesicular or dyshydrotic reaction of the sole often appears in patients suffering for months or years with interdigital tinea pedis. Vesicles or vesicopustules are seen near the instep and on the mid anterior plantar surface. This vesicular reaction may be limited. Vesicles may rupture, leaving a fine collarette scaling and then heal spontaneously. When new vesicles appear, the clinical aspect of healing and vesicular lesions can take an eczematous appearance.

- **Ulcerative Type:** It is associated with maceration, weeping, denudation and ulceration. Secondary maceration with overgrowth of the bacterial flora commonly complicates the eruption, leading to an inflammatory "mixed" process (complex type). Generally, ulceration in the web space with secondary bacterial infection occurs in the immunocompromised patients with interdigital tinea pedis.

8. TINEA UNGUIUM

Synonyms: Onchomycosis

Invasion of the nail by a dermatophyte is referred to as tinea unguium, whereas onychomycosis is derived from a Greek word onyx (nail) and mykes (fungus), which is the invasion of the nail by any fungus, including dermatophytes as well as non-dermatophyes. Toenails as well as fingernails can be infected, but toenails are more often affected, probably owing to the warm and moist environment of the shoes, as well as trauma. T. rubrum accounts for 70% of all cases while T. mentagrophytes var. interdigitale for 20%. On rare occasions, other species are involved.

Onychomycosis can occur at any age, although it is more common with increasing age. It is uncommon before puberty or in normally menstruating women. Males and females are equally affected. Immunosuppression, hyperhidrosis, diabetes mellitus, and decreased vascular supply with aging are other factors responsible for this type of infection.

- **Distal Lateral Subungual Onychomycosis:** This is the most common type and accounts for a little more that 90% cases of tinea unguum. The fungus invades the distal and lateral borders of the horny layer of the hyponychium and/or the distal nail bed. The infection then moves proximally to invade the ventral surface. This causes thickening of the horny layer, raising the free edge of the nail plate, which may be followed by onycholysis. The subungual debris also provides a site for secondary infection by bacteria or other moulds and yeast. Discoloration ranges from white to brown.

- **Endonyx Onychomycosis:** It has been described only recently as a rare type of onychomycosis. The infection, which is due to T. soudanensc, is clinically characterized by a diffuse milky-white discoloration and the absence of nail bed hyperkeratosis or onycholysis.

- **Superficial White Onychomycosis:** It is also known as leukonychia mycotica or leuconychia trichophytica. It is the second most common type of onychomycosis.

It is normally confined to the toenails and T. mentagrophytes var. interdigitale is responsible for more than 90% of the cases. Recently T. rubrum has been reported as an infrequent cause. Apart from these, Fusarium oxysporum, or species of Aspergillus or Acremonium are also reported. This type differs from the other variants by primarily invading the dorsal surface of the nail plate. In the beginning, white patches with distinct edges, away from the free edge of the nail on the dorsal nail plate, are seen, but they can coalesce and eventually cover the whole nail. The surface becomes rough and the texture softer than normal.

- **Proximal Subungual Onychomycosis:** This is an unusual type of finger and/or toenail onychomycosis. The infection begins in the proximal nail fold. When it reaches the matrix, the fungus, usually T. rubrum, invades the lower portion of the nail plate and a white spot appears under the cuticle which advances distally.

- **Total Dystrophic Onychomycosis:** It represents the most advanced form of onychomycosis. The nail crumbles and disappears, leaving a thickened, abnormal nail bed retaining keratotic nail debris. In AIDS patients, this evolution can go rapidly and start as a proximal subungual onychomycosis.

DERMATOPHYTID/"ID REACTION"

The immune mechanism in Dermatophytosis may lead to the appearance of secondary rashes at a site distant from the site of the associated dermatophyte infection, called id reaction. It accounts for 4-5% of cases of Dermatophytosis. It may be due to the local immunologic response to systemically absorbed fungal antigens.[136] However, in one series of dermatophytids, only half had a positive reaction to trichophytin. The lesions are mycologically negative, but secondary bacterial infection may occur. The onset is at times accompanied by fever, anorexia, generalized adenopathy, spleenomegaly, and leukocytosis. These reactions tend to occur at the height of dermatophyte infections, slightly thereafter, or just after the initiation of systemic antifungals. Clinically it may take several forms, including follicular papules, erythema nodosum, vesicular id of hands and feet, erysipelas-like, erythema annularre centrifugum, and urticaria. The most common of these is a type of acute vesicular eczema or pompholyx that occurs on the hands and feet in patients with inflammatory ringworm of the feet, mainly caused by T. mentagrophytes. Disappearance of the id lesions occurs after a successful treatment of Dermatophytosis, but every now and then topical or systemic steroid therapy along with antifungals is warranted, especially if the dermatophytid is extremely widespread or inflammatory.

DIFFERENTIAL DIAGNOSIS

There are certain diseases that mimic the diagnosis of Dermatophytosis and therefore be differentiated from the similar presenting diseases.

Table 2: Differential Diagnosis of Tinea Infections.

Differential Diagnosis of Tinea Infections		
Infections	Causative Species	Differential Diagnosis
T. Capitis	Trichophyton.tonsurans Microsporum .audouinii Zoophilic Microsporum .canis*	Alopecia areata, Impetigo, Pediculosis, Psoriasis, Seborrheic dermatitis, Traction alopecia, Trichotillomania
T.Corporis	Trichophyton.rubrum Epidermophyton.floccosum	Cutaneous lumps erythematous, Eczema, Psoriasis, Erythema multiforme, Granuloma annularre, pityriasis rosea, Nummular eczematous dermatitis, Secondary syphilis, Drug eruption, Tinea (pityriasis) versicolor
T. Cruris	T. rubrum E. floccosum T. mentagrophytes	Candidal intertrigo, Contact dermatitis Erythrasma, Psoriasis, Seborrhoea
T.Manuum	T. rubrum	Same as with tinea pedis
T. Pedis	T. rubrum E. floccosum T. mentagrophytes	Bacterial or candidal infection, Contact or atopic dermatitis, Dyshidrosis, Eczema, Psoriasis, Pitted keratolysis
T.Unguium	T.rubrum T. mentagrophytes	Contact dermatitis, Lichen planus Onychodystrophy, Psoriasis

QOOBA (DERMATOPHYTOSIS)

Differential diagnosis of tinea capitis includes alopecia areata, seborrheic dermatitis, psoriasis, trichotillomania, bacterial folliculitis, and cicatrical alopecia.

Seborrheic dermatitis usually occurs in older children and does not cause hair loss. Lack of scaling is typical of alopecia areata and usually trichotillomania. Alopecia areata causes circumscribed areas of hair loss but does not scales and the "exclamation mark" hairs seen in this condition – broken hairs tapering from the fractured end toward the skin surface – are pathognomonic.

Tinea barbae should be distinguished from sycosis barbae, actinomycosis, folliculitis, pyoderma and granulomas. In sycosis barbae, there is chronic congestion of skin of the beard region with superficial, follicular pustules. Actinomycosis produces a hard, indurated, lumpy swelling below the angle of jaw.

Tinea corporis should be differentiated from discoid eczema, impetigo, psoriasis, lupus erythematosus, erythema annularre centrifugum, pityriasis rosea, erythema multiforme, secondary syphilis, Granuloma annularre, erythema chronicum migrans, sarcoidosis.

The important points to look for the annular scaling margins of lesion and follicular prominence. In eczema active inflammatory border will be absent and there will be bilateral symmetrical patches, usually on limbs and appears in winter. Psoriasis has typical silvery and distributed over elbow, knee, scalp and nails. The candle grease sign will be present. Secondary syphilis is often manifested by characteristic palmer, plantar and mucous membrane lesion. Erythema multiform does not have peripheral scales, is mostly acral in distribution, and is often associated with herpes simplex. Tinea corporis rarely has the long numbers of lesion seen in pityriasis rosea. Granuloma annularre lacks scales.

Tinea faciei must be differentiated from seborrheic dermatitis, discoid lupus, roasacea, contact dermatitis and polymorphic light eruption.

Tinea cruris differentiation includes interriginous candidiasis, Erythrasma, psoriasis, eczematous dermatitis, intertrigo, Seborrheic dermatitis.

In candidiasis of the groins, the lesions are moist, deep red, with some typical satellite pustules. There is no central clearing and increased inflammation of the borders and the scrotum is commonly affected. In erythrasma which is caused by Corynebacterium minutissimum, the lesions are uniform in color, red to brown, and there is no scaling or central clearing. The borders are sharply demarcated, but not infiltrated. Intertrigo tends to be more red, less scaly and presents in obese individuals in moist body folds with less extension on to thigh. Seborrheic dermatitis of inguinal area also often involves the face, sternum and axilla. Flexural psoriasis has no resemblance to tinea cruris, except that it occurs on the same site; lesions of psoriasis are present on other areas of the body as well.

Tinea pedis differential diagnosis includes erythrasma, candidiasis, psoriasis, dyshidrosis, contact dermatitis, palmoplanter pustulosis, syphilis keratoderma, arsenic drug eruption.

In the differential diagnosis of dyshydrotic lesions, atopic or allergic contact dermatitis and hyperhidrosis with pitted keratolysis must be excluded. Pustular lesions must be differentiated from pustular psoriasis or palmoplantar pustulosis. An acute inflammatory vesicular tinea pedis may be accompanied by a vesicular, allergic reaction (mycide reaction) of the hands. This pompholyx-like reaction is only seen in severe, acute inflammatory tinea.

Chronic tinea pedis must be differentiated from chronic eczema and psoriasis. In children, one must consider the possibility of juvenile plantar dermatosis. In this disease, the skin is dry, chapped and often fissured. The contact surface of the big toe and the weight-bearing parts of the sole and heel are affected. Chronic tinea pedis is rare in children. In hyperkeratotic forms, a differential diagnosis with hereditary keratosis palmoplantaris must be made.

Tinea manuum should be differentiated from psoriasis, contact dermatitis, eczema, pityriasis rubra pilaris, Irritant and allergic dermatitis of the hands or palmer psoriasis are much more common than tinea manus and are typically bilateral. The presence of finger nail Onychomycosis would be a clinical clue of tinea manuum and would help differentiate it from psoriasis, eczema, contact dermatitis, and pityriasis rubra pilaris.

Tinea unguium, the differential diagnosis includes candidiasis, lichen planus, psoriasis, bacterial infection, contact dermatitis, traumatic onychodystrophies, paronychia congenital, nail bed tumours, yellow-nail syndrome, idiopathic onycholysis, moniliasis, syphilis, Reiter syndrome.

Nail plate is typically covered with fine pits and/or small salmon colored droplet on the plate evident of psoriasis of nail. Candida infections of the nail begin in the proximal nail plate and are associated with nail fold infection but toe nail infection is rare.

Lichen planus can be differentiated by looking for the violaceous purple papules on the extremities or by other signs on the mucous membranes. Hardness of nail plate, its increased longitudinal curvature and the light green/yellow are all typical in yellow nail syndrome. If the onycholytic nail is clipped to allow examination of the nail bed, the latter will be normal if the symptom is caused by trauma rather than Onychomycosis.

LABORATORY DIAGNOSIS

There are no. of ways by which dermatohytosis can be diagnosed; investigations specifically employed for the diagnosis of Dermatophytosis are described below:

1. Direct microscopic examination:

Direct examination is essential as it allows the clinician to start treatment pending culture.

- **Skin scraping:** In skin scraping the first step is to obtain material by gently scraping at the margins of the lesion with a scalpel. Glass slide can also be used for scraping. If the lesions have vesicles or bullae, the tops of the vesicles or bullae should be clipped and included in the sample, as the greatest number of organisms are found in the roof of the blister. Suppurating lesions may be sampled with a swab when it is impractical to obtain scrapings. Other skin dermatohytosis, such as tinea pedis and tinea manuum, are scraped in such a way that the whole infected area is represented, since an advancing margin is often not evident. If there is minimal scaling, sellotape can be used to collect material for examination. The strips of sellotape are placed with the sticky side down on a glass slide. The sample obtained is mounded on a glass slide and one to two drops of 10 or 20% KOH (potassium hydroxide) are added. KOH helps to dissolve the keratin, but the fungal filaments resist this treatment as they have a chitinous wall. Some staining methods often involve the addition of a drop of Parker Quink stain or any other blue/black fountain pen ink. Next, a glass cover slip is placed over the mount. The cover slip is pressed gently to crush the scales. The slide is then allowed to stand for 15-20 minutes to clear the sample. Finally it is examined under the microscope, first in low power, followed by high power. The mycelium may be seen under low power, but better observation of both hyphae and spores is obtained by the use of reduced illumination. True hyphae are seen as long, hyaline, branching, often septate rods or uniform width. Spores may be seen as small spherical bodies lying singly or in the clusters. Cotton fibers, cell borders and other artifacts may be falsely interpreted as possible findings. According to some reports, KOH examination is positive in only one third patients. As keratin is rapidly digested by KOH, an immediate examination is required. This limitation may be overcome by the use of Amann's chloral-lactophenol which allows clearing without heating. It is helpful when direct examination is differed, and it is particularly recommended for examination and conservation of hair samples. Other dissociating agents have also been proposed; including 10% sodium hydroxide (NaOH) and detergents. Xylol is as satisfactory as KOH and need not be warmed. A rapid staining method using 100mg of chlorazol black E in 10ml of dimethyl sulfoxide (DMSO) and adding it to 5% aqueous solution of KOH can be helpful. Congo red can also be used for direct examination.

- **Examination of hair:** The scalp is first examined under filtered ultraviolet light (Wood's Lamp). Hair roots and crusts will be plucked from the infected area or its edge, particularly when these elements are glowing under UV lamp and suppurating lesions will be swabbed. Hair is best sampled by plucking so that the root in included. If this is not possible due to hair fragility, as in 'black dot' tinea capitis, a scalpel may be used to scrape the scales and excavate small portions of the hair roots. Brushes with stiff bristles run firmly across the lesion have also been used successfully to sample T. capitis. The rest of the procedure is similar to skin scraping.

- **Examination of nails:** In the case of distal subungual onychomycosis, samples are usually obtained, after nail clipping, by scraping with a small curette or a scalpel blade from the lower nail table, particularly at the edge of the lesion. Indeed, viable fungal hyphae may be encountered only near the nail bed. Nail specimens are slow to clear. Therefore, the full thickness nail clippings may be placed in a weak (5%) KOH solution kept in a watch glass for 24 hours to obtain adequate clearing. The presence of septate hyphae under the microscope confirms the diagnosis of tinea.

2. Culture

Culture needs to be done when the KOH mount is negative or when it is necessary to identify the fungal species. The most common medium used for isolating dermatophytes is Sabouraud's dextrose agar (SDA). Various formulations of this medium are commercial available; some have additives that inhibit bacterial and non dermatophyte growth. A dermatophyte test medium (DTM) indicator can also be used. DTM is an alternative medium devised by Taplin et al. It contains antibiotics (gentamicin sulphate and chlortetracycline HCL), an agent to control saprophytic fungi (cycloheximide) and penol red indicator. It normally shows alkalinity generated by dermatophyte growth as the color changes from yellow to red.

After the affected area has been cleansed with 70% alcohol, scraping is done with the usual technique. The material so obtained is inoculated on the surface of the medium. It is kept at 26C and examined every alternate day. No culture should be discarded unless kept for three weeks.

Macroscopic examination: It includes the examination of colony surface for growth rate, color, texture and topography. Examination of the reverse of the colony to characteristic pigment is also done.

Microscopic examination: It includes the examination of arrangement of spores, types of hyphal appendages and hyphal modification. Further examination can be done after staining with lactophenol cotton blue. Urease test and slide culture can also be employed.

Characteristic of some common pathogenic species in culture;

a. Trichophyton rubrum

Colony morphology: mounded white centre, maroon reverse pigment, urease negative

Microscopic: Few tear shaped microconidia, pencil shaped macroconidia, hair perforation negative.

b. Trichophyton mentagrophyte

Colony morphology: white to creamy with a cottony, mounded surface, no reverse pigment, urease positive.

Microscopic: Clustered round microconidia, rare cigar shaped macroconidia, occasionally spiral hyphae. Hair perforation positive.

c. Microsporum audouinii

Colony morphology: flat and white to grey with widely spaced grooves, tan to salmon reverse pigment.

Microscopy: Terminal chlamydoconidia and pectinate hyphae.

d. Epidermophyton floccosum

Colony morphology: Flat feathery colonies with a central fold and yellow to dull grey green pigment.

Microscopy: No microconidia, numerous thin and thick walled club shaped macroconidia.

3. Skin Biopsy

Skin biopsy is done when diagnosis of a dermatophyte infection remains in question after office testing or failure to respond to treatment. Sample is collected from a fully developed primary lesion. Involuting lesions or secondarily infected lesions should not be selected. Fungal staining with periodic acid-Schiff (PAS or Hotchkiss Mc Manus) stain shows purple red color and highlights fungal elements when examined under the microscope. Grocott-Gomori methenamine-silver (GMS) stain can also be used. Hematoxylin and Eosin (H&E), though not commonly used for staining fungus, is regarded as the best stain for studying tissue response to etiologic agents. Other stains which can be used are alcian blue, Mayer's mucicarmine and Gridley fungus (GF) stains.

4. Wood's light examination

The UV (ultraviolet) rays are thrown on the scalp in a dark room and any florescence noted. It may be falsely negative in around 50% of cases. Bright green florescence is seen in ectothrix infection caused by M. canis, M. audouinii and M. ferruginem. A dull green florescence is seen in favus caused by T. shoenleinii.

5. Newer Techniques

- Polymerase chain reaction enzyme analysis.

- Immunoperoxidase staining.

- Dual flow cytometry.

- In vivo confocal microscopy.

MANAGEMENT

Unani Treatment

In Unani treatment of Qooba is directed mainly according to the causative substances, i.e., akhlat (humours), clinical presentation, severity and duration of the disease. Unani medicine follows the principle of nuzj-wa-istifragh, which aims at Tanqiya-e-badan. In the majority of cases Qooba occur due to deranged sauda. So, in most of the instances, treatment is aimed at removal of sauda from the body. The drugs having the effects of tahleel, taqtee and talteef are also used for ghaleez maadda (thick morbid matter). For haar and raqeeq maadda (hot and thin morbid matter), drugs having the property of taskeen and tarteeb are used. In addition to oral therapy, there is a treasure trove of efficacious topical drugs and formulations, which are frequently advised. Apart from this, some tadabeer (regimental therapies) are also advised in the treatment of this disease.

Ibn-e-Sina advised taleeq (leech therapy), hammam (bathing) and dietary recommendation, providing moist and wet environment, and avoiding dryness. Ibn-e-Sina held taleeq (leeching) better than drug therapy. According to him hammam is also a good option for treatment. Leeching was also advised by various other scholars like Zakaria Razi. Fasd (venesection) and Hijamat bil shurt (wet cupping) has also been found to be beneficial by Unani Scholars.

Treatment According to dominating khilt:

Jins-e-Damvi: Fasad (venesection) is performed at a nearest possible site for the removal of morbid matters. Ghassal (detergent) advia should be applied locally.

Tila: The following drug combinations in the form of paste are advised topically.

Kharpaza, Ushna, Arad Baqla and arad Nakhood.

Samagh Arabi, Samagh Farsi, Ushq and vinegar.

Application of Roghan-e-Gandum is also indicated. Leeching can be done if these regimens fail.

Jins-e-Ratubi: Matbookh Aftimoon (decoction) and Ayarij Fiqara for the removal of morbid fluid is used.

Gargle: Decoction of Maveezaj, Aqarqarha in honey water

Tila: The following drug combinations, in the form of paste, are advised topically.7 Aqlimia zahab and Hartal should be ground in Gulnar and Gul-e-surkh, mixed into vinegar.

Aspand, Kandash, Turbud ground and mixed with vinegar.

Grounded Asafetida root mixed with vinegar can be massaged over the affected area. Also, the saliva and the tartar of a fasting person may be applied locally.

Jins-e-Saudavi: This is the worst among all the types of Qooba, and it does not respond easily. Therefore, removal of morbid saudavi matter is essential. Use of matbookh aftimoon and laughazia with aab-e-halela siyah and zabeeb is indicated for the same. Fasd (venesection) of vareed-e-basleeq (basilica vein) is also indicated.

Tila: Wax, fats of ducks and cocks should be applied regularly.

Treatment depending on the morphology of the disease:

If the disease is acute, superficial and localized, local application is usually enough, e.g., roghan-e-gandum, roghan-e-alsi, roghan-e-badam talkh, roghan-e-narjil, butter and ghee. Wax mixed with kateera and sibr can also be used as tila.

If the disease is at a stage where it has penetrated beyond the skin into the muscles, then relatively more potent drugs like ushq mixed with vinegar should be applied after leeching.

QOOBA (DERMATOPHYTOSIS)

If the disease is chronic and situated in deeper tissues, then the management is started with the removal of morbid saudavi matters from the body by fasd (venesection) and ishal (purgation). For local application very potent drugs which are haad and muhammir, such as hartal and khardal, are used until fresh bleeding occurs. After this, healing is facilitated by the use of appropriate drugs. Hijamat bil shurt (wet cupping) over the lesion and hammam are also indicated in this stage.

Some formulations for local application by eminent Unani scholars are:

- Vinegar + ushq/ radish seeds9/ rasot/ murmuki/ asafetida/ hummas/ samaghe arbi/ zaravand mudharraj/ roghan-e-badam talkh.
- Vinegar + roghan-e-gandum + zaravand + zarnikh + ushq + muqil + khardal + zaj.
- Vinegar + cinnamon + honey.
- Honey + Chuqandar water/ garlic/ suddab.
- Ushq + nakchikni + henna.
- Lemon juice + opium + ard singhara.
- Sulphur + kundur + zaj + sibr + samagh-e-arbi.
- Sulphur + tukhm-e-shadnaj/ ilakul batam.
- Sulphur + kat safed + sugar + opium.
- Curd + sabus gandum + olive oil.
- Zafat romi + mom zard

    Some compound drugs for local applications with specific names are

- Habb-e-Qooba (Plaspapra, sulphur, borax, opium, lemon water)

- Habb-e-Daad (Sublimed sulphur, camphor, guggul, aloe vera, borax)

- Marham-e-Daad (Sublimed sulphur, kasis, alum, bitter almond)

- Marham-e-Zararih (Telini fly, ghee)

- Marham-e-Qooba (Ilkul batam, ushq, muqil, zaravand, rose oil, goat fat, bee was)

- Roghan-e-Qooba (Kamela oil, neem oil, curd)

Modern Treatment

In the allopathic system of medicine use of topical and systemic antifungal agents is the mainstay for the treatment of Dermatophytosis. The choice of treatment and its duration depends on the causative organism, the site of infection, the extent of the disease, chronicity, concurrent disease and medication. Topical therapy alone is generally effective for an uncomplicated and localized T. corporis, T. cruris, T. faciei, T. manuum and limited T. pedis. For local application keratinolytics are used along with antifungals. Some indications for the systemic therapy of dermatophyte infections are extensive skin infections, skin infections failing to respond to appropriate topical therapy, scalp infections, majocchi's granulomas, and onychomycosis with multiple nails involved.

Table 3: Treatment of Dermatophytosis.

Treatment of Dermatophytosis	
Clinical Pattern	**Treatment**
Tineapedis Interdigital	Topical cream/ointment: terbinafine, imidazoles (micinazole, econazole, clotrimazole etc.) undecenoic acid, tolnaftate.
Dry type	Oral: terbinafine 250 mg/day for 2-4 weeks, itraconazole 400 mg/day for 1 week/month (repeated if necessary), fluconazole 200 mg weekly for 4-8 weeks.
Tinea Corporis Small lesion	Topical cream/ointment: terbinafine, imidazole (micinazole, econazole, clotrimazole etc.)
Large lesion	Oral: terbinafine 250 mg/day for 2 weeks, itraconazole 200 mg/day for 1 week, fluconazole 250 mg weekly for 2-4 weeks.
Tinea Capitis	Griseofulvin: 10-20 mg/day for minimum 6 weeks Terbinafin:< 20 Kg: 62.5 mg/day; 20-40 kg: 125 mg/day;> 40 Kg: 250 mg/day. Itraconazole: 4-6 mg/kg Pulsed dose weekly. Fluconazole: 3-8 mg/kg pulsed dose weekly.
Tinea Unguium Finger nail	Terbinafine: 250 mg/day for 6 weeks Itraconazole: 400 mg/day for 1 week each month, repeated for 2-3 month Fluconazole: 200 mg/week for 8-16 weeks
Toe nail	Terbinafine: 250 mg/day for 12 weeks Itraconazole: 400 mg/day for 1 week each month, repeated for 2-4 months. Fluconazole: 200 mg/week for 12-24 weeks

PREVENTION AND CONTROL

Prevention and control of dermatophyte infections must take into consideration the area invaded, the etiologic agent, and the source of infection. Routine inspection of scalps of young children should be performed at the beginning of the school term. Good hygiene should be impressed upon those infected, and they must be instructed not to share headgear, combs and brushes. All those infected must be treated promptly to prevent further spread of the infection.

Although nosocomial spread of Dermatophytosis is rare, a few outbreaks have been reported. Such outbreaks must be investigated promptly to avoid further spread.

Since tinea corporis and tinea cruris caused by Anthropophilic fungi which can be transmitted by infected clothing, towels, and bedding, these should be disinfected after use and infected individuals should not permit others to share them.

It is important to locate the animal reservoir in infections caused by the zoophilic dermatophytes. Good hygiene and sanitation and fungicidal sprays and washes have been effective in controlling these infections.

Prevention of tinea pedis may be enhance by using good foot hygiene (includes regular washing of the feet, thorough drying, and application of foot powder); avoiding excessive moisture and occlusion by wearing sandals or other well-ventilated shoes; avoiding trauma to the feet, especially blistering by ill-fitting footgear; and not sharing towels, socks, or shoes.